Diabetes and Me: A Simple Guide to Understanding Your Disease

Dr. Ebony N. Raymond D.O.

Copyright © 2019 Dr. Ebony N. Raymond D.O.
All rights reserved.
ISBN: 9781652547587

For inquiries write to:
The Medical Institute for Wellness
Dr. Ebony Raymond D.O.
3105 W 15th St.
Suite E
Plano, TX 75075

Scripture taken from the NEW AMERICAN STANDARD BIBLE®, Copyright © 1960,1962,1963,1968,1971,1972,1973,1975,1977,1995 by The Lockman Foundation. Used by permission."

DEDICATION

To Dr. Chris Rheams D.O. our beloved Program Director who always believed in me more than I did. Thank you for always giving me cart blanche to execute my ideas and for putting up with all of my crazy dreams! Sir, you are truly the physicians' physician and an amazing leader. Thank you for all of your sacrifice.

To Dr. and Mrs. Deme and Lydia Gurmu M.D. without your love and support, I would never have made it through residency. Words cannot express my gratitude for you both and your precious family.

To Dr. Tanisha Hayes D.O. without your support I would definitely have quit medical school!

CONTENTS

	Introduction...	5
1	**Chapter 1: Diabetes Basics**..	7
	What is Diabetes?..	7
	Nutrition 101...	7
	How Diabetes Occurs..	8
	Diagnosis of Diabetes...	9
	Test Your Knowledge Chapter 1.......................................	10
	Test Your Knowledge Answer Key Chapter 1....................	11
	Wellness Corner..	12
2	**Chapter 2: Management and Treatment of Diabetes**...............	14
	Healthy Diet...	14
	Treatment Options...	15
	Insulin Therapy...	19
	Treatment Goals..	21
	Glucose Monitoring...	22
	Test Your Knowledge Chapter 2.......................................	23
	Test Your Knowledge Answer Key Chapter 2....................	24
	Wellness Corner..	25
3	**Chapter 3: Complications of Diabetes**................................	29
	How Your Disease Affects You...	29
	Prevention and Treatment of Complications.....................	32
	Test Your Knowledge Chapter 3.......................................	34
	Test Your Knowledge Answer Key Chapter 3....................	35
	Wellness Corner..	36
4	**Chapter 4: Meal Planning and Weight Loss**........................	38
	The Importance of Weight Loss in Diabetes......................	38
	Nutrition 201...	38
	Test Your Knowledge Chapter 4.......................................	45
	Test Your Knowledge Answer Key Chapter 4....................	47
	Wellness Corner..	48
	Endnotes..	51
	References...	52
	Glossary..	53
	Appendix...	55
	About the Author...	62

INTRODUCTION

So, either you or a loved one have recently been diagnosed with diabetes, and you have no idea what to do next, right? Well you have definitely come to the right book. This book is a brief and simple guide to understanding your disease. As a physician, I have found that diabetes is one of the most difficult subjects for patients to understand. In fact, proper treatment of the disease is a difficult topic for physicians in training to understand! You are not alone. The problem with diabetes is that when it is not treated and managed properly, it can negatively impact your health and quality of life. Plus, patients have an important role in managing their disease apart from just taking medications. Knowledge gives you the tools to do so. Also, according to studies, most of the reading material that we give patients in clinic is too difficult to understand. While this book is not a substitute for proper evaluation and treatment by your physician, I hope that it makes the subject matter easier to understand thus, making your disease more manageable. Each chapter contains knowledge about diabetes, a quiz to test yourself on the information that you just learned, and a wellness corner section to show you how you can apply the knowledge presented. At the end of the book there are glucose monitoring logs to assist you along your journey as well as a glossary of terms to help with the definitions of some of the confusing and scary words associated with diabetes. It is my sincerest hope that by learning more about the disease process, it takes away the fear and uncertainty about you or your loved one's recent diagnosis.

Be well!

-Dr. Ebony N. Raymond D.O.

---

*The content in this book is not intended to be a substitute for professional medical advice, diagnosis, or treatment. Always seek the advice of your physician or other qualified health provider with any questions you may have regarding a medical condition.

CHAPTER 1: DIABETES BASICS

What is Diabetes?

Diabetes is a metabolic disorder that involves high sugar (glucose) levels also known as hyperglycemia. In simple terms, diabetes is a condition where the body cannot process sugar. This condition can lead to several problems that affect your overall health and quality of life. Diabetes is typically grouped into two types: Type 1 and Type 2. But first, in order to understand what diabetes is, we have to understand the basics of nutrition and the role of glucose or sugar in the body.

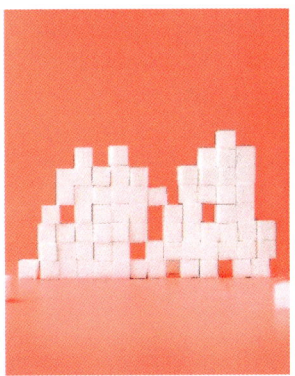

Nutrition 101

Food is made up of 3 major building blocks: carbohydrates, protein, and fat. There are 3 main types of carbohydrates in food: starches, sugars, and fiber. Examples of starches include vegetables such as peas, corn, and potatoes as well as beans, and grains such as oats, rice, and barley. These are known as complex carbohydrates. Sugars are known as simple carbohydrates and consist of two types: Single sugars (or monosaccharides) known as fructose (found in fruit), glucose, and galactose. The second type are double sugars (or disaccharides) known as lactose (found in milk), sucrose (table sugar), and maltose. Fiber is the part of plant foods that cannot be absorbed and aids in gut health.

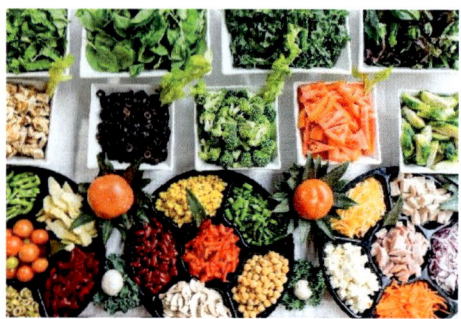

<u>How Diabetes Occurs</u>

Your Pancreas and Insulin

The pancreas, an organ located near the stomach is part of your digestive system. When you eat a meal that contains carbohydrates, the body breaks them down into glucose (also known as sugar but for the rest of the book we will simply say glucose). The pancreas then releases insulin in response to the arrival of glucose. Insulin allows the glucose to be taken up and used for energy to the cells of muscle and the brain. Diabetes is a condition where the glucose is not properly taken up by insulin. Either insulin is absent, or it is not enough for the amount of glucose that has been eaten. These differences help to determine if a person has Type I or Type II diabetes.

Type I Diabetes

Is described as an autoimmune disease. It is largely a genetic disorder (may run in the family) but environment may also play a role. Autoimmune disease means that the body attacks the cells of the pancreas that release insulin and destroys them. This results in a pancreas that cannot make insulin. As a result, glucose cannot be used by the cells leading to a build-up of glucose called hyperglycemia (too much glucose) and the breakdown of fat tissue for energy. It is typically diagnosed in children and teens.

Type II Diabetes

Is described as disorder of "insulin resistance". Both genetics and environment play a role with the greatest factor being extra weight or obesity. Lack of exercise and poor diet leads to the pancreas working harder to release more insulin to take extra glucose into the cells. Over time, the pancreas cannot keep up and hyperglycemia occurs.

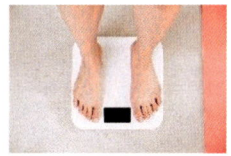

Pre-diabetes

Patients that are overweight or obese with poor diet and little activity are at high risk for developing diabetes in the future. Often times these patients are pre-diabetic. Prediabetes is a condition where the glucose levels are high due to insulin resistance but not high enough to be classified as diabetes. A diagnosis of prediabetes is a chance to make lifestyle and diet changes before becoming diabetic. Studies show that losing just 10-15lbs can prevent one from developing diabetes in the future.

Diagnosis of Diabetes

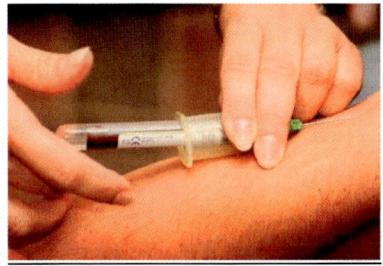

A simple blood test done in your doctor's office can show that you have diabetes. A fasting (at least 8 hrs. or more without food before testing) glucose level greater than 126 at least twice confirms the diagnosis. HgbA1c (glycated hemoglobin) may also be used. This measurement can be done with a simple fingerstick in the office or a lab test. It is the average glucose level over the past 3 months. A HgbA1c of 6.5% and greater confirms the diagnosis of diabetes. Lastly, if a glucose sample is drawn randomly (not fasting) and is 200 or greater with the patient experiencing increased urination, hunger, or thirst, this automatically indicates diabetes and does not require repeat testing.

A diagnosis of prediabetes is confirmed by a fasting glucose between 100-125 and a HgbA1c between 5.7-6.4%

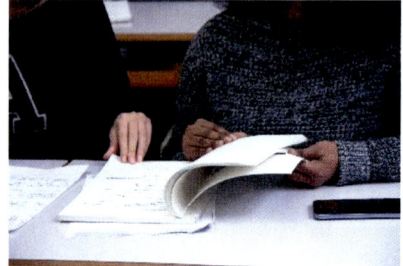

Test Your Knowledge Chapter 1

1) Diabetes is caused by high _____ levels.
   a. Protein
   b. Fat
   c. Carbohydrate
   d. Glucose

2) Type 1 Diabetes is caused by _____
   a. Eating too much sugar
   b. Not enough physical activity
   c. Genetics
   d. Destruction of the pancreas
   e. Both C and D

3) The 3 major components of food include:
   a. Fat, Protein, and Lipids
   b. Fat, Protein, and Carbohydrates
   c. Carbohydrates, Fat, and Fiber
   d. Fat, Starch, and Carbohydrates

4) Type II Diabetes is caused by:
   a. Genetics
   b. Environment
   c. Destruction of the pancreas
   d. A and B
   e. All of the above

5) The greatest risk factor for developing Type II Diabetes is:
   a. Obesity
   b. Lack of exercise
   c. Poor diet
   d. All of the above

Test Your Knowledge Answer Key

1) D

2) E

3) B

4) D

5) D

Wellness Corner: Start Improving Your Health Today

We will discuss treatment as well as meal planning in the next few chapters. However, today you can start to make small changes that will improve your diabetes. First you can start to incorporate exercise into your daily activities. The President's Council on Sports, Fitness, and Nutrition recommends that adults should do at least 150 minutes to 300 minutes a week of moderate-intensity, or 75 minutes to 150 minutes a week of vigorous-intensity aerobic physical activity, or an equivalent combination of moderate- and vigorous-intensity aerobic activity. Preferably, aerobic activity should be spread throughout the week. Adults should also do muscle-strengthening activities of moderate or greater intensity and that involve all major muscle groups on 2 or more days a week.[i]

If you did 30 minutes of walking at a fast pace 5 times a week, you would complete the 150 minutes recommended. Or you can do longer exercises fewer times a week.

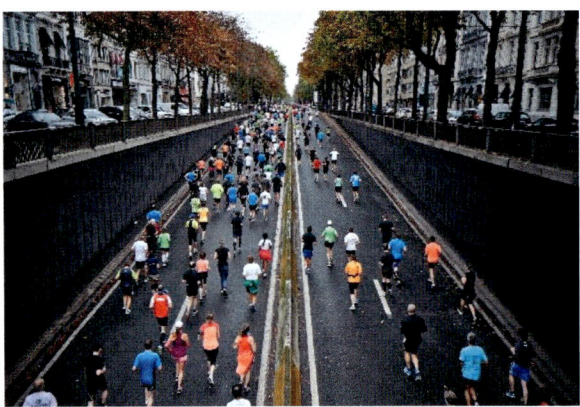

There are several simple ways to increase your activity level:

1) Increase your steps. Using a pedometer start off slowly and aim for a goal of 10,000 steps daily.

2) Join a local gym and attend group fitness classes if available.

3) Take the stairs instead of the elevator.

4) Visit your local park and start walking at least 30 minutes/day most days of the week.

The second change you can make is with diet. As we continue our discussion on nutrition, you will learn more and be able to make better choices concerning the food that you eat. However, today you can make a change by simply cutting out processed foods and simple sugars. What does this mean? Instead of chips, candy, or soda replace with whole foods such as veggies, lean meats, and some fruit in small portions.

Steps to a better you.
First list your height and weight to calculate your BMI and most recent HgbA1c (if available).

Height_____ inches

Weight_____ lbs.

BMI_____ (weight/height^2) x703) For example if you are 5'3 and weigh 184 lbs., then you BMI will= (184lbs/63inches^2) x703 **32.59**

HgbA1c_____%

We will later discuss BMI, goal setting, and weight loss so we will revisit these numbers to track progress.

Now, list 3 things that you can do today to change:

1) _____

2) _____

3) _____

Chapter 2: Management and Treatment of Diabetes

Healthy Diet

One of the most important parts of managing your diabetes is eating a well-balanced diet. As we discussed in the first chapter, food is made up of fat, carbohydrates, and protein. A well-balanced diet is one that consists of all three in moderate amounts. The average American diet typically includes about 50-60% of carbohydrates. Below is a basic breakdown of these building blocks or macronutrients of the food that we eat.

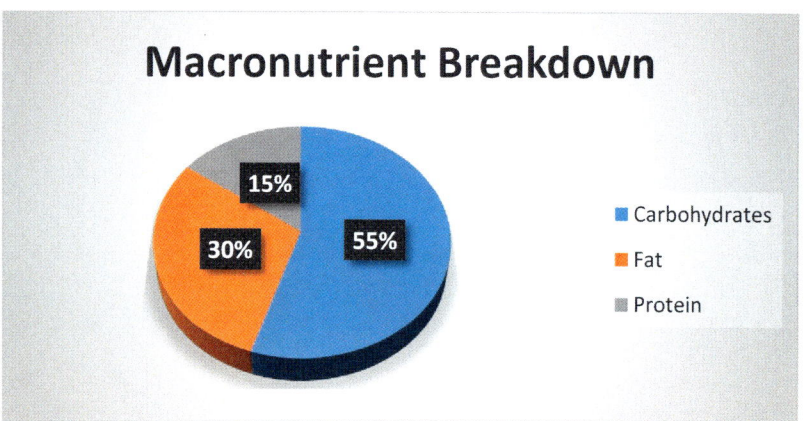

Glycemic index

As we discussed in Chapter 1, there are 3 main carbohydrates in food including starches, sugars, and fiber. However, not all carbohydrates are the same. Some foods can raise your glucose more than others. The glycemic index (also known as GI), measures how a food containing carbohydrate raises glucose levels. We will discuss meal planning, how to read nutrition labels, and carbohydrate counting in the final chapter but for now we will discuss basic meal planning with the GI. For the diabetic patient, it is important to choose foods that have a low or medium GI. This means that the particular food eaten will not cause glucose levels to rise as

Low GI Foods	Medium GI Foods	High GI Foods
<ul><li>100% stone-ground whole wheat</li><li>Oatmeal (rolled or steel-cut)</li><li>Barley</li><li>Sweet potatoes, corn, beans</li><li>Most fruits, non-starchy vegetables and carrots</li></ul>	<ul><li>Whole wheat, rye, and pita bread</li><li>Quick oats</li><li>Brown, wild, or basmati rice, couscous</li></ul>	<ul><li>White bread</li><li>Corn flakes, puffed rice, bran flakes, instant oatmeal</li><li>White rice, pasta, macaroni and cheese from mix</li><li>White potatoes</li><li>Snack foods such as pretzels, chips, crackers</li><li>Melons and pineapple</li></ul>

high as they would if you ate pure sugar. The table above indicates the type of foods grouped from low to high GI.

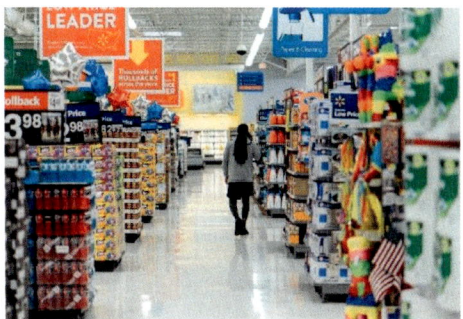

Treatment Options

We discussed in Chapter 1 the differences between Type I and Type II diabetes. Since Type I diabetes is caused by destruction of the cells in the pancreas that make insulin, the treatment is always insulin. However, in Type II diabetes, the treatment depends on many factors. When a patient has a diagnosis of pre-diabetes, the treatment options may include a period where the patient will try to control glucose levels by exercising, weight loss, and eating a better diet. For Type II diabetics that have been recently diagnosed, most patients are given Metformin (also known as Glucophage) by their doctors. Metformin is a pill that is usually taken one to two times daily. It works by decreasing the ability of the body to produce glucose and makes the cells more sensitive to insulin. The most common side effects that patients have are diarrhea and/or nausea and vomiting. Typically, these side effects stop after a few weeks. Below is a list of the most common medications used for treatment of Type II diabetes and the most common side effects

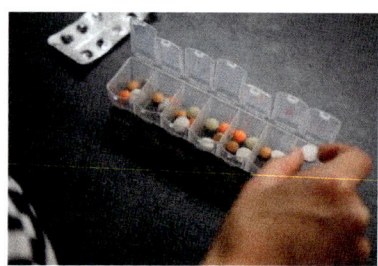

Drug Class	Drug Name (Generic and Brand)	How it Works	Common Side Effects	Special Things to Consider
Sulfonylureas	Glimepiride (**Amaryl**), Glipizide (**Glucotrol**), Glyburide (**Dia Beta, Micronase**, or **Glynase**)	Causes the pancreas to release insulin	Low blood sugar (hypoglycemia) Weight gain	Cannot be used in Type I Diabetics or long-term Type II Diabetics because requires active cells in pancreas to release insulin
Meglitinide Analogs	Repaglinide (**Prandin**)	Causes the pancreas to release insulin (similar to sulfonylureas)	Low blood sugar (hypoglycemia) Weight gain	N/A

Drug Class	Drug Name (Generic and Brand)	How it Works	Common Side Effects	Special Things to Consider
D-Phenylalanine Derivative	Nateglinide (**Starlix**)	Causes the pancreas to release insulin (similar to sulfonylureas)	Low blood sugar (hypoglycemia) Weight gain	N/A
Biguanides	Metformin (**Glucophage**)	Stops the production of glucose	GI side effects (nausea, vomiting, diarrhea) Lactic acidosis	Cannot be used in patients with severe kidney disease
Thiazolidinediones	Pioglitazone (**Actos**), Rosiglitazone (**Avandia**)	Increases the sensitivity of the tissues to insulin	May cause leg swelling (edema)	Avandia has been shown to increase possibility of developing heart disease including heart attack Cannot be used in patients who have heart failure
Alpha-Glucosidase Inhibitors	Acarbose (**Precose**)	Stops enzymes from breaking down starch and sucrose	Abdominal bloating and gas Diarrhea	When combined with insulin or sulfonylureas can cause low blood sugar
GLP-1 Receptor Agonists	Dulaglutide (**Trulicity**), Exenatide (**Byetta** or **Bydureon**), Liraglutide (**Victoza**), Semaglutide (**Ozempic**)	Slows digestion, helps decrease breakdown of stored glucose (also known as glycogen)	May cause modest weight loss (1-6 lbs.) May decrease appetite Nausea and Vomiting Diarrhea	May Increase risk of pancreatitis Cannot be used in patients with medullary thyroid cancer or MEN (multiple endocrine neoplasia) syndrome Type II

Drug Class	Drug Name (Generic and Brand)	How it Works	Common Side Effects	Special Things to Consider
DPP-4 Inhibitors	Linagliptin (**Tradjenta**), Saxagliptin (**Onglyza**), Sitagliptin (**Januvia**)	Slows digestion, helps decrease breakdown of stored glucose (also known as glycogen), increases insulin release	Increase in upper respiratory infections	Rarely may cause allergic reaction such as skin rash or difficulty breathing which is a medical emergency
SGLT2 Inhibitors	Canagliflozin (**Invokana**) Dapagliflozin (**Farxiga**) Empagliflozin (**Jardiance**)	Decreases the amount of glucose that is reabsorbed back into the body and releases into the urine.	May cause increase in urinary tract infections	Cannot be used in patients with kidney disease

May increase LDL levels (bad cholesterol) May decrease bone density leading to fractures |
| *Miscellaneous* | Coesevelam (**Welchol**)

Pramlitide (**Symlin**) | Welchol

Symlin decreases appetite, slows digestion, and decreases breakdown of stored glucose (also known as glycogen) | Welchol can cause constipation and indigestion

Symlin can cause hypoglycemia and nausea | Welchol may increase triglyceride levels Symlin can be used in patients with Type I DM |

Insulin therapy

As discussed in Chapter 1, over time, Type II diabetics that have had the disease for several years may no longer produce insulin. As a result, these patients will need to be placed on insulin. Also, patients that have a HgbA1c of 10% or greater at time of diagnosis or patients that are diagnosed during hospitalization for a life-threatening condition known as DKA (we will discuss later in chapter 3), also need to be started on insulin because pills may not lower the glucose levels enough. However, these patients with a new diagnosis of diabetes may be able to stop insulin and start on pills if the glucose is better controlled after a few months.

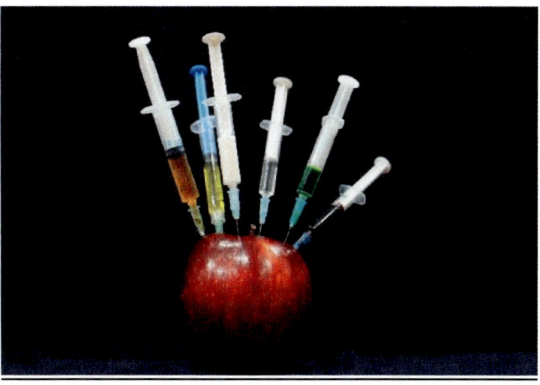

There are 5 types of insulin that are grouped by how quickly they act on the body and for how long as shown in the table below. These groups include rapid acting, short acting, intermediate, premixed, and long acting. Rapid acting and short acting are typically taken before meals. Intermediate and pre-mixed are usually taken twice daily; in the morning and at night. Long acting is typically taken at bedtime, but some patients take it in the morning or at morning and bedtime.

Type of Insulin	Name of Insulin	How quickly it acts	How long it lasts
Rapid acting	Lispro (**Humalog**), Aspart (**Novolog**), Glulisine (**Apidra**)	5-15 minutes	3-4 hours
Short acting	Regular insulin Inhaled regular insulin (**Afrezza**)	30-60 minutes	6-8 hours
Intermediate acting	**NPH**	2-4 hours	10-20 hours
Premixed	Consists of NPH with a rapid acting insulin		
Long acting	Glargine (**Lantus, Toujeo, Basaglar**) Detemir (**Levemir**) Degludec (**Tresiba**)	0.5-1.5 hours	17-42 hours

Some patients with difficult to control blood sugar (especially Type I diabetics) are often prescribed insulin pumps. Insulin pumps have the ability to deliver basal (long acting insulin) and bolus (pre-meal or short acting insulin). The settings are typically tailored for the patient by an endocrinologist (a diabetes specialist). However, for the purpose of this book, we will not go further in detail on this subject.

There are different ways to inject insulin. One of the most common ways it to use syringes. When using this method, the insulin is in a vial which is a small glass container that holds a liquid medication. The medication is drawn up using a syringe which has a needle at the end to inject the insulin. Some insulins come in a pen form that can be easier to use for those who are unable to draw up insulin from the vials on their own.

When injecting insulin, you should inject in areas covered by loose skin. The most common area used is the stomach. Other areas include the thigh and upper arms. It is important to rotate the areas that you inject as injecting at the same site daily can result in visible lumps or small dents in the skin (a condition called lipodystrophy).

Risk Factors of Insulin Therapy

Low blood sugar also known as hypoglycemia, is the most common problem in patients that inject insulin. However, as we see in our study of oral medications earlier, some pills can also cause low glucose levels. Symptoms typically occur when the glucose levels fall to about 60 or below and include sweating, racing heart, and nausea. If not treated quickly, symptoms can worsen to include confusion, vision loss, fainting, seizure, and ultimately death. Therefore, it is important for patients to be able to quickly recognize the symptoms of low blood sugar and know how to correct it. Diabetic patients should carry glucose tablets or juice at all times. A good rule of thumb is that low glucose levels can be corrected with 15 grams of carbohydrate which can include a piece of candy, tablespoon of sugar, or a cup of juice/soda. You may also speak with you doctor about prescribing an emergency injection kit called glucagon that can raise your blood sugar quickly.

<u>Treatment Goals</u>

Once you have been started on either medication, insulin, or both, you doctor may want to see you more regularly until your glucose levels are controlled. In order to determine whether the medicine is helping to lower your blood sugar levels appropriately, your doctor will go by certain guidelines. For instance, the ADA (American Diabetic Association) recommends patients achieving a HgbA1c of 7.0% or less.[ii] These guidelines also include having a fasting blood sugar between 80-130 and a reading of less than 180 two hours after meals. The after-meal glucose reading is also called a post-prandial glucose. The American Association of Clinical Endocrinologists have stricter guidelines including a HgbA1c of 6.5% or less, a fasting glucose of less than 110 and a reading of less than 140 two hours after meals.[iii] Discuss with your doctor concerning treatment goals for your particular situation.

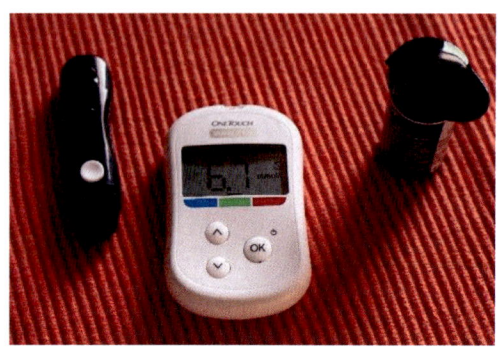

<u>Glucose monitoring</u>

Glucose monitoring by a device called a glucometer, is typically only needed for those using insulin therapy. However, sometimes your doctor may want you to monitor your blood sugar levels closely if you have problems with low blood sugar our if your HgbA1c is consistently high. Glucometers are small and can be taken anywhere. Along with the glucometer, you will also need lancets and test strips. The lancet is used to prick your finger to get a blood sample. The blood is then placed on the test strip which is read by the blood glucose monitor. How often you check your blood sugar will depend on what your doctor recommends and the type of therapy he/she has prescribed. Typically, if you are using both long and short acting insulin, the glucose is checked fasting when you first get up in the morning, before meals, and sometimes 2 hours after meals.

There are also continuous glucose monitoring systems such as the DexCom or FreeStyle Libre. These systems use a sensor instead of a fingerstick multiple times a day like the traditional glucometer. In addition, it monitors your blood sugar throughout the day and the information can be sent to a smartphone or other devices.

At the end of this chapter and the back of the book, are glucose monitoring logs. This allows you to keep track of your glucose at various times of the day along with the food eaten. This is how you can begin to see how certain foods affect your blood sugar and learn over time which foods to avoid.

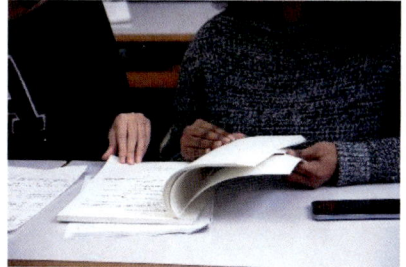

Test Your Knowledge Chapter 2

1) The glycemic index is a measure of the_____ of carbohydrate eaten.
   a. Amount
   b. Calories
   c. Glucose
   d. Type

2) What is a common complication of insulin therapy?
   a. Hunger
   b. Hypoglycemia
   c. Dizziness
   d. Diarrhea
   e. Vomiting

3) What is the most common medication used for Type II diabetes?
   a. Insulin
   b. Actos
   c. Trulicity
   d. Metformin

4) Type I diabetics are always prescribed insulin.
   a. True
   b. False

5) The treatment goal for all diabetic patients is a HgbA1c of what level?
   a. 7.5% or less
   b. 8% or less
   c. 7% or less
   d. 10% or less

Test Your Knowledge Answer Key

1) D

2) B

3) D

4) A

5) C

Wellness Corner: Start Improving Your Health Today

As you begin to change your diet and watch what you eat more carefully, there are a few tips that you can keep in mind while grocery shopping, eating out, and planning meals. These tips take the glycemic index into consideration as it is important to remember that certain foods will affect your blood sugar more than others. Overall, you still have to think about how much food you are eating and making sure that you are eating a well-balanced diet from all of the major food groups. Here are 3 tips to help you on your journey to eating better.

1) The GI of a food only describes the type of carbohydrate that you are eating. For instance, if you have a low GI food such as steel-cut oatmeal for breakfast, portion sizes still matter. (Just because it is low GI doesn't mean that it is carbohydrate free, it still affects your blood sugar just not as poorly as other foods).

2) When grocery shopping on a whim or eating out without this guide, just remember that food higher on the glycemic index will be items that are more processed (typically fast foods items; think French fries, tacos, or store-bought baked goods such as pie).

3) The GI of a food is different when eaten alone vs being eaten with other foods. When eating a high GI food, you can combine it with other low GI foods to balance out the effect on your glucose. For example, you can eat brown rice which has a medium GI with black beans that are low on the GI. Or you can have pineapple which is high on the GI with steel-cut oatmeal which has a low GI.

In summary, when grocery shopping, try to choose whole grains and whole foods such as fruit and vegetables instead of processed foods like chips, cereal, and white bread.

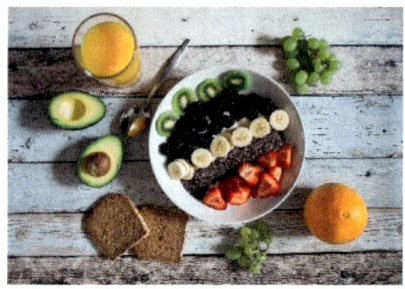

Steps to a better you
Now, list 1 food that you can give up starting today that you now know is not good for you. In addition, list 2 more foods that are good for you that you can start including in your diet.

1)
_____

2)
_____

3)
_____

      Below is a sample glucose monitoring log. You can record the date, your glucose, time of day, and food eaten when glucose was checked. When you visit your doctor, you can share this log and he/she can make changes to your medication or diet if necessary. There are more sheets available at the end of the book in the appendix.

Glucose Monitoring Log

Date	Fasting Glucose	2 Hour After Breakfast Glucose	Before Lunch Glucose	Before Dinner Glucose	Bedtime
Example 1/1/20	90	180 **Breakfast:** Oatmeal, 1 banana, 2 slices of bacon	160 **Lunch:** Burrito bowl with chicken and black beans	200 **Dinner:** Salmon, baked potato with sour cream, Steamed veggies	250 **Snacks:** candy bar, 1 can of soda

Date	Fasting Glucose	2 Hour After Breakfast Glucose	Before Lunch Glucose	Before Dinner Glucose	Bedtime

Chapter 3: Complications of Diabetes

<u>How Your Disease Affects You</u>

The reason that diabetes is such an important topic is because it has an impact on nearly every major organ system in your body. What this means is that diabetes ultimately begins to affect your heart, blood vessels, eyes, nerves, skin and so much more. These effects may happen sooner rather than later the more uncontrolled your disease is. The chances of suffering these effects are also higher the longer you have diabetes. The American Diabetic Association states that in 2015, Diabetes was the 7th leading cause of death in the United States.[iv] These are heartbreaking statistics and the key to improving them is to make sure that you the patient, have all of the tools that you need to manage your disease.

Also, when glucose levels are too high, patients can develop a serious condition called DKA which requires being treated in the hospital in the intensive care unit. If not addressed and treated quickly, it can result in death. Now we will talk about individual complications by the particular organ that they affect.

Vision complications

Diabetes is the leading cause of blindness between the ages of 20 and 74 in the United States.[v] This loss of vision is caused by diabetic retinopathy (disease of the retina). The retina allows us to recognize objects and our loved ones by sensing light and sending that information to our brains.

There are 2 types of retinopathy: non-proliferative and proliferative. We will not go into great detail on the differences. However, the basic information needed to know is that over time if blood sugar levels are always elevated, it starts to cause changes in the blood vessels of the eye. As this continues, it begins to affect the blood flow to the retina. This is non-proliferative retinopathy. If not corrected, the retina does not have enough blood supply (a condition called retinal ischemia). The body then responds by making new blood vessels. However, the new blood vessels begin to appear near other important parts of your eye (i.e. macula and optic nerve). These new vessels can easily rupture which can cause bleeding and in worst case scenario, detachment of the retina. This is proliferative retinopathy. These changes to the eye can be seen by an ophthalmologist (a doctor that specializes in disease of the eyes).

Kidney complications

The kidneys are so important to our overall health. The kidneys work to filter harmful things from our body, help control our blood pressure, assist with making red blood cells, and make sure that our electrolytes are in balance. High blood sugar levels can damage our kidneys and cause a condition known as diabetic nephropathy (disease of the kidney). This diabetic nephropathy can lead to severe disease called ESRD (end-stage renal disease) where a person needs machines to help rid the body of harmful toxins because the kidneys no longer work. This is called dialysis.

Damage to the kidneys from diabetes takes a long time and you will not know that you have kidney disease until it becomes severe. Kidney disease can be seen by testing the amount of protein in the urine. Healthy kidneys do not allow protein to spill out into the urine so if protein is there, this shows that damage has occurred. This test can be done by giving a urine sample.

Nerve complications

Diabetic neuropathy (disease of the nerves) can be found in about 50% of people with Type I or II diabetes who have had the disease for several years.[vi] If your nerves are affected, you may have numbness, tingling, or burning in the legs or feet. At night you may feel as if pins and needles are stabbing your legs. As the nerve damage continues, you may lose the ability to feel in your feet and your muscles may weaken over time. This becomes dangerous because when you lose feeling, you can stub your toe or step on something sharp and develop a wound that you may never see. Severe wounds on the foot if not treated quickly can result in a loss of your foot/leg. This is why it is so important for diabetic patients to check their feet daily for sores/wounds and to wear shoes that protect them from hurting their feet.

Heart complications

Studies show that heart disease is increased in those with diabetes. Also, diabetic patients with heart disease often have worse outcomes than patients without diabetes. High glucose levels along with obesity, high cholesterol, and high blood pressure increase the rate and chance of a diabetic having heart disease. In addition, diabetic patients may have "atypical" or "silent" chest pain (not the classic chest pain most people feel when having a heart attack), making detecting signs of a heart attack more difficult.

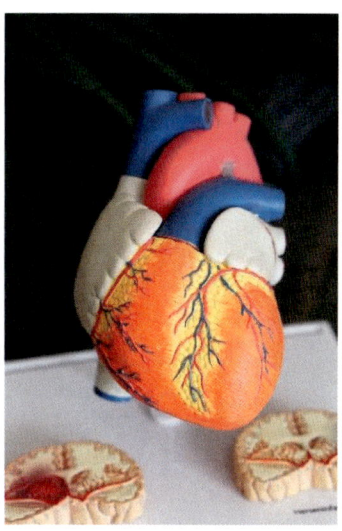

Risk of infections

Diabetic patients are more likely to have infections. These infections may include urinary tract infections (UTI), pneumonia, and skin infections. Some of the most common skin infections include cellulitis (caused by bacteria) and yeast infections. The more uncontrolled the blood sugar, the more likely you may be to develop these infections. In addition, diabetic patients are also at a higher risk to develop an infection after surgery.

DKA/HHS

DKA and HHS are serious life-threatening conditions that are caused by severely high glucose levels. Glucose levels can be as high as 600 or more. DKA (diabetic ketoacidosis) and HHS (hyperglycemic hyperosmolar state) are very similar except for a few differences. DKA is typically seen in Type I diabetics and symptoms usually occur over a 24-hour time period. These symptoms may include nausea and vomiting, stomach pain, and shortness of breath. DKA can be caused by infection, heart attack, and/or lack of regularly taking your insulin. HHS is typically seen in Type II diabetics. Unlike DKA, symptoms occur gradually over a few weeks and symptoms can include weight loss, increased urination, and confusion. It is typically caused by a serious infection or illness in addition to lack of proper water intake over time.

Prevention and Treatment of Complications

For all complications related to diabetes the number one key to prevention is better control of your blood sugar. In chapter 1, we talked about treatment goals of glucose levels and HgbA1c. Weight loss, taking your medications as prescribed, and eating a healthy diet will help you to reach those goals. Listed below are more ways to prevent and treat the most common complications of diabetes.

Diabetic Retinopathy

One of the best ways to prevent eye disease is to visit an ophthalmologist every year. Most diseases of the eye found in diabetic patients can be treated if detected early. If, however advanced proliferative retinopathy is already present, eye injections and laser therapy are usually able to prevent complete vision loss.

Diabetic nephropathy

Proper control of blood pressure will help to either prevent or stop the progression of kidney disease. Your doctor may also prescribe a blood pressure medication known as an ACE inhibitor (such as Lisinopril) or an ARB (such as Losartan) as it protects the kidneys as well as helps with blood pressure. If the kidney function continues to get worse, your doctor may send you to a nephrologist (kidney specialist). When the kidneys are close to not working properly anymore, you may be referred for a kidney transplant and or dialysis depending on your age and other health conditions.

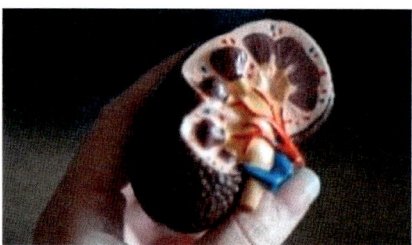

Diabetic neuropathy

Treatment of nerve pain typically includes medications. The most common medications used are antidepressants. These medications include Cymbalta, Elavil, or Nortriptyline. Other medications used include Lyrica, and Gabapentin. Sometimes, patients may need to see a pain management doctor if their symptoms are severe. In addition, because of the danger that we talked about earlier of developing wounds on the feet without knowing due to loss of feeling, it is recommended that diabetic patients see a podiatrist (foot doctor) regularly in addition to checking their feet every night.

Heart disease

Treatment of heart disease in the diabetic patient is similar to that of a non-diabetic patient. It includes cholesterol lowering medications called statins, ACE inhibitor or ARB as we discussed earlier for blood pressure control, and heart surgery for those with severe disease. The ADA also recommends that patients who are high risk for heart disease take an aspirin daily to prevent complications. High risk patients include those greater than 50 years old, and other risk factors including high blood pressure, high cholesterol, smoking, and family history. [vii]

DKA/HHS

Prevention of DKA and HHS would include making sure that you take your insulin and other diabetic medications as prescribed and being treated for infections sooner rather than later. Treatment involves admission to the hospital typically in the intensive care unit. Since patients are dehydrated as well, they are given IV fluids as well as continuous IV insulin.

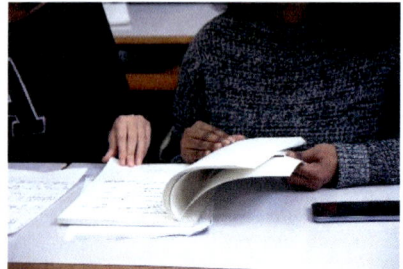

Test Your Knowledge Chapter 3

1) A life-threatening complication of diabetes known as _____ requires a hospital stay and IV insulin.
   a. BKA/HHH
   b. Hyperglycemia
   c. DKA/HHS
   d. Hypoglycemia

2) Diabetic nephropathy is a complication of diabetes that affects_____
   a. Nerves
   b. Kidneys
   c. Heart
   d. Skin

3) Diabetic neuropathy is a complication of diabetes that affects_____
   a. Nerves
   b. Kidneys
   c. Heart
   d. Skin

4) Diabetes is one of the leading causes of vision loss in the United States.
   a. True
   b. False

5) What type of doctor does a diabetic patient need to see yearly for eye exams?
   a. Podiatrist
   b. Nephrologist
   c. Ophthalmologist
   d. Endocrinologist

Test Your Knowledge Answer Key

1) C
2) B
3) A
4) A
5) C

Wellness Corner: Start Improving Your Health Today

As a diabetic patient, there are a few things that you can do starting today other than managing your glucose to prevent some of the complications that we discussed earlier in the chapter.

1) Schedule an eye exam every single year. A lot of diabetic patients don't think that this is an important part of managing their disease, but it is. As we discussed earlier, an eye specialist can see changes in the eye earlier preventing vision loss in the future.
2) If you already have nerve damage from diabetes, you MUST check your feet every night. In addition, you should see a podiatrist every year. Also, it is good to invest in diabetic shoes for extra protection and decrease the risk of developing a serious wound.
3) Since diabetics are more likely to get certain infections, make sure that you are up to date with all of your vaccines by talking with your doctor.
4) If you have other risk factors for developing complications such as smoking, high blood pressure or high cholesterol, do everything in your power to stop smoking and take all of your medications just like the doctor prescribed them.

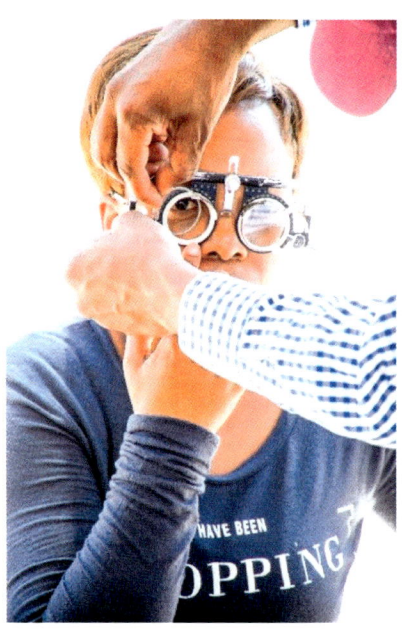

Steps to a better you.
List 2 ways that you have not helped prevent complications from diabetes. (It may be not taking your medicine regularly, smoking, or not visiting the doctor regularly) Now, list 1 thing that you will do starting today to improve you bad habits.

1) _____

2) _____

3) _____

Chapter 4: Meal Planning and Weight Loss

<u>The Importance of Weight Loss in Diabetes</u>

Losing weight is one of the most important things that you can do to help manage your disease. In fact, when patients are newly diagnosed and become committed to their health and start to lose weight, their disease process can be reversed. They may not even need to take medications, just continue exercising and living a healthy lifestyle. However, one of the most common questions that I get from patients is "How do I lose weight?" And this is a valid question because majority of the diabetics have Type II diabetes and have spent most of their life eating poorly and not getting enough physical activity. This chapter will help answer that question and be your guide on your journey to a better and healthier you!

<u>Nutrition 201</u>

In chapter 1, we talked about basic nutrition including the building blocks of food. Now we will go into more detail. Every single piece of food that we eat has a value to it called a calorie. A calorie is a unit of energy. In the most basic definition of weight loss, weight loss happens when we put out more energy than we take in. Thus, we have to burn more calories than we eat. And this is the problem with majority of the people that want to lose weight. The typical American diet and lifestyle is one where we eat way too much because of large portion sizes, and we do not exercise enough to burn off what we eat. This leads to weight gain. Now in order to determine a healthy weight for you, we will look back at the end of chapter 1 where you calculated your BMI. Below is a chart to see the classification of weight status based on your BMI. Take note that as the BMI increases, so do the health and diabetes risks.

BMI	Weight Classification
<18.5	Underweight
18.5-24.9	Normal Weight
25.0-29.9	Overweight
30-34.9	Obesity (Class I)
35-39.9	Obesity (Class II)
40 and up	Obesity (Class III)

Now this is where it may get a little difficult but please stay with me! (For those of you who hate math, please don't get angry lol!) These are the equations that we use to calculate ideal body weight.

The example that I will use here is a woman that is 5'6 (or 66 inches) and 190 lbs.

I will use the equation below to calculate ideal body weight for a woman. 45.5 kg +2.3kg (66 inches-60inches) =**286.8 kgs.** We will then convert kgs to lbs. by dividing 286.8 kgs/2.20462= **130 lbs.** Therefore, the ideal body weight for a female that is 5'6 is 130 lbs.

- Ideal body weight (IBW) (men) = 50 kg + 2.3 kg x (height in - 60)
- Ideal body weight (IBW) (women) = 45.5 kg + 2.3 kg x (height in - 60)
- To convert kgs to lbs., divide the amount in kgs/ 2.20462

Now we will calculate the new BMI using the ideal body weight of 130 lbs. BMI= (weight/height^2) x703) For example using our 5'6 tall patient and now 130 lbs. for weight, the new BMI is= (130 lbs./66inches^2) x703 ~**21.** This patient is now at a healthier weight from the old BMI which was **30.6.**

Calories count

Now that we know our ideal body weight, it is important that we take the number of calories that we eat daily into consideration. This is important because you can clean up your diet and start exercising but if you continue to eat too much, you will not lose weight.

There are a few basics to calorie counting. 1lb of fat= 3500 calories. A healthy weight loss is typically 1-2 lbs. every week. In order to do that, we must have a deficit of 500 calories for 7 days which equals 3500 calories. (This means that we need to eat 500 calories less every day to lose 1 lb. a week) In order to do that we can combine eating less AND exercising. Now there are more calculations to help you determine how many calories you should eat daily based on weight, height, and activity level. However, I will not punish you with any more math for the rest of the book! Below are tables from the United States Department of Health to help you estimate the number of calories needed every day.[viii] These tables are divided by male and female and are grouped according to age and exercise level. If you do not currently exercise or have a job where you do not perform any activity all day, your activity level will be sedentary. Moderately active and active are based on job activity and exercise level.

For this example, let's use a 35-year-old male that does not exercise. Based on the table below, his average calorie intake is 2400 calories if he wants to stay the same weight. If he wants to lose 1 lb. every week, he must cut 500 calories per day from his diet. In order to do this, he may cut 300 calories from his diet and exercise for 30 minutes every day burning 200 calories resulting in a total loss of 500 calories per day. Because he changed his diet and added exercise, he is now getting 1900 calories per day.

MALES

AGE	Sedentary[a]	Moderately active[b]	Active[c]
15	2,200	2,600	3,000
16	2,400	2,800	3,200
17	2,400	2,800	3,200
18	2,400	2,800	3,200
19-20	2,600	2,800	3,000
21-25	2,400	2,800	3,000
26-30	2,400	2,600	3,000
31-35	2,400	2,600	3,000
36-40	2,400	2,600	2,800
41-45	2,200	2,600	2,800
46-50	2,200	2,400	2,800

MALES

AGE	Sedentary[a]	Moderately active[b]	Active[c]
51-55	2,200	2,400	2,800
56-60	2,200	2,400	2,600
61-65	2,000	2,400	2,600
66-70	2,000	2,200	2,600
71-75	2,000	2,200	2,600
76 and up	2,000	2,200	2,400

FEMALES[d]

AGE	Sedentary[a]	Moderately active[b]	Active[c]
15	1,800	2,000	2,400
16	1,800	2,000	2,400
17	1,800	2,000	2,400
18	1,800	2,000	2,400
19-20	2,000	2,200	2,400

FEMALES[d]

AGE	Sedentary[a]	Moderately active[b]	Active[c]
21-25	2,000	2,200	2,400
26-30	1,800	2,000	2,400
31-35	1,800	2,000	2,200
36-40	1,800	2,000	2,200
41-45	1,800	2,000	2,200
46-50	1,800	2,000	2,200
51-55	1,600	1,800	2,200
56-60	1,600	1,800	2,200
61-65	1,600	1,800	2,000
66-70	1,600	1,800	2,000
71-75	1,600	1,800	2,000
76 and up	1,600	1,800	2,000

For those of you that did not quite get the equations earlier, this is much easier and is simple to do daily. When first starting out, it can be quite easy to cut out extra calories. Often times when I discuss weight loss with patients and go over the foods that they eat, many love soda and other sugary drinks (i.e. fancy coffee drinks). One 20 oz bottle of soda is about

240 calories and very high in sugar. A small frappe or latte from your favorite coffee shop can easily contain 300 calories or more! This really hurts your diet when you drink more than one every day. Just cutting out one bottle of soda or sugary coffee drinks daily will help you on your weight loss journey.

Nutrition labels

Now that you understand a little more about calorie counting, we will now discuss how to read nutrition labels. This is important as reading nutrition facts can help you keep your portion sizes smaller and will allow you to see just what you are putting into your body. Below is a sample nutrition label provided by the U.S. Department of Health.[ix]

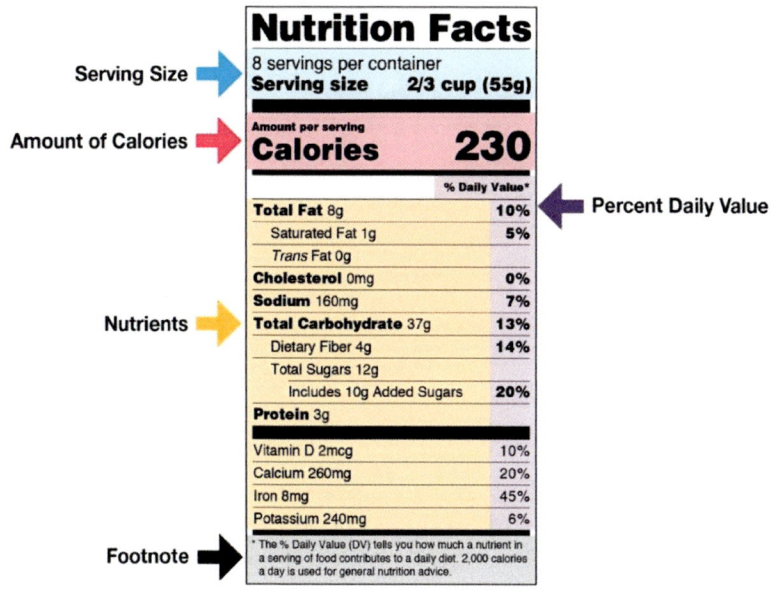

(For educational purposes only. These labels do not meet the labeling requirements described in 21 CFR 101.9.)

From the label there are several important things to pay attention to when reading. The first is the serving size. Since one of the most common problems people have when trying to lose weight is overeating, the serving size should be one of the first things that we look at. Second, we look at the number of servings per container. Some people make the mistake of looking at the nutrition facts thinking that it is for the entire package, but we see that there are 8 serving per package. Third, we look at the number of calories per serving. Fourth, we look at the nutrients including our food building blocks: fat, protein, and carbohydrates. Lastly, we look at the ingredients which are not featured on this sample label but will be on almost every food item that you purchase. Remember from chapter 1 the glycemic index. When reading the ingredient list just remember that the more processed the product is (i.e. if it contains high fructose corn syrup and a lot of ingredients that you cannot pronounce) the higher it is on the glycemic index and you should avoid it or not eat it often.

So, let's put all of this information together as we look at our nutrition label again. Let's say that this label is for a bag of rice. The serving size is 2/3 cup. No need to break out the measuring cup, this is roughly about the size of your fist and each serving is 230 calories, 8 g of fat, and 37 g of carbohydrates. But let's say that you are still hungry and get a second helping. You have now eaten 460 calories, 16 g of fat, and 74 g of carbohydrates.

Portion control

Controlling the amount of food that you eat should not be hard or take a lot of guess work. To be able to estimate portion and serving sizes, you can compare to everyday objects. For instance, 1 serving of vegetables is 1 cup and is about the same size of a baseball. One serving of fruit is similar to the size of a tennis ball or computer mouse. A portion of meat such as steak, fish or chicken is 3 oz; about the size of the palm of your hand or a deck of cards. 1 tablespoon of peanut butter or salad dressing is about the size of your thumb. If you keep these simple things in mind, you will have no problem controlling portion sizes.

Carbohydrate counting

As we learned in chapter 2, carbohydrates make up about 50% of the typical American diet. Other health professionals and nutrition experts give a recommended daily intake of about 45-65% of our diet coming from carbohydrates or at least 130 g daily. This just means that about half of what eat will be carbohydrates. However, these are recommendations for the general population not diabetics. The ADA recommends that each individual eat the amount of carbohydrates that are best for their body and lifestyle.[x] In general, glucose control will be better with fewer carbohydrates. Therefore, since most diabetics typically ate more than the recommended amount prior to being diagnosed with diabetes, about 45-50% or at least 130 g daily of carbohydrates is a good starting point to aim for. Keep in mind that glucose is important for brain energy so eating too few carbohydrates can cause lower energy levels and weakness. Speak with your doctor about how many carbohydrates you should be eating daily.

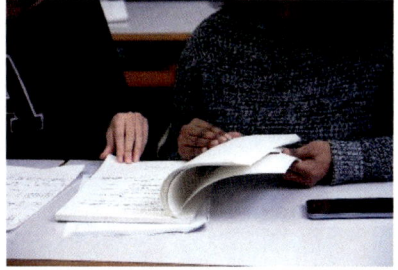

Test Your Knowledge Chapter 4

1) A _____ measures the amount of energy that is in a food.
   a. Gram
   b. Calorie
   c. Carbohydrate
   d. Serving size

2) Based on the nutrition label above, how much is one serving size?
   a. 4 servings
   b. 46 grams
   c. 2 cups
   d. 1 ½ cup

3) Based on the nutrition label above, how many grams of carbohydrates are in 2 serving sizes?
   a. 46 grams
   b. 7 grams
   c. 92 grams
   d. 4 grams

4) In order to lose weight, you have to burn more calories than you eat.
   a. True
   b. False

5) How many calories are in 1 lb. of fat?
   a. 3,500 calories
   b. 5,000 calories
   c. 2,500 calories
   d. 3,000 calories

Test Your Knowledge Answer Key

1) B
2) D
3) C
4) A
5) A

Wellness Corner: Choosing Smart Meals

You now have all of the tools that you need to make good decisions when it comes to choosing healthy meals. We will compare a day of eating a typical diet vs healthier meal options.

HEALTHIER OPTION	**TYPICAL DIET**
Breakfast:	**Breakfast:**
½ cup steel-cut oats Handful of almonds ½ cup skim milk Raisins 1 tablespoon brown sugar	2 pancakes with butter and syrup 2 slices of bacon 1 glass of orange juice 2 eggs
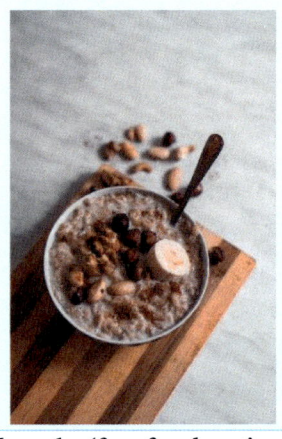	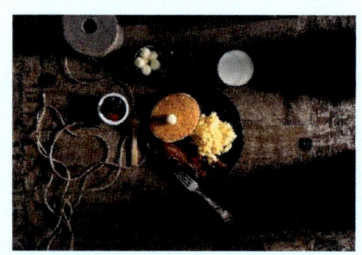
Lunch: (fast food option) Burrito bowl with: Grilled chicken breast Brown rice Black/pinto beans Salsa Veggies	Lunch: (fast food option) Cheeseburger Fries Ice cream
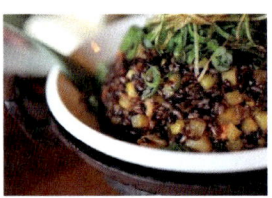	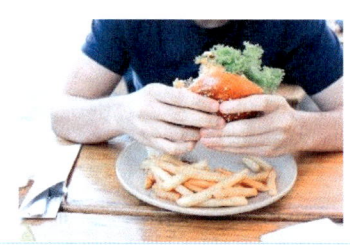

Dinner:
Baked salmon
Sautéed broccoli
Side salad with 2 tablespoons of Italian dressing (without croutons or cheese, all veggies)

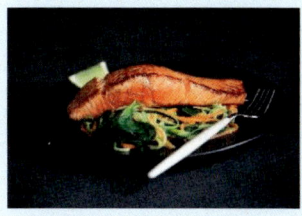

Snack: 1 container of fruit-flavored Greek yogurt

Dinner:
Fried fish
Baked potato with butter, cheese and sour cream
Caesar side salad

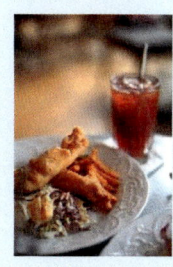

Snack: 1 bag of chips and 20 oz bottle of soda

Total nutrition facts:
Breakfast: 375 calories, 6.5 g fat, 14 g protein, 56.4 g carbohydrates

Lunch: 570 calories, 14.5 g fat, 45 g protein, 67 g carbohydrates

Snack: 120 calories, 0 g fat, 12 g protein,
18 g carbohydrates

Dinner: 562 calories, 34 g fat, 44 g protein, 20 g carbohydrates

Grand total
1627 calories, 55 g fat, 115 g protein, 161 g carbohydrates

Total nutrition facts:
Breakfast: 830 calories, 35 g fat, 29 g protein, 104 g carbohydrates

Lunch: 720 calories, 27 g fat, 23 g protein, 92 g carbohydrates

Snack: 390 calories, 9 g fat, 2 g protein, 80 g carbohydrates

Dinner: 961 calories, 59 g fat, 46 g protein, 60 g carbohydrates

Grand total
2901 calories, 130 g fat, 100 g protein, 336 g carbohydrates

As you can see the healthier options have less calories, fat, and carbohydrates. Also, the carbohydrates in the healthier meal plan are lower on the glycemic index. Keep in mind that this is just a guide. There are so many different foods to choose from. In addition, the food from the typical diet meal plan are not all bad. While they should not be eaten often, they can still be eaten on occasion with smaller portion sizes. The goal is to improve your diet by having more balance not trying to eat perfectly. If you begin to apply everything that you have learned so far to your everyday life, you will begin to see improvement in your glucose readings, energy levels, and overall health.

Steps to a better you.

Since you know what a healthy meal plan looks like, try to keep a track of everything that you eat over the next week. This is really easy and quick to do. There are several apps that you can download if you have a smart phone. They will allow you to record your food and calculate your nutrition facts like we did above. This will let you see just how much you are eating daily and how you can improve.

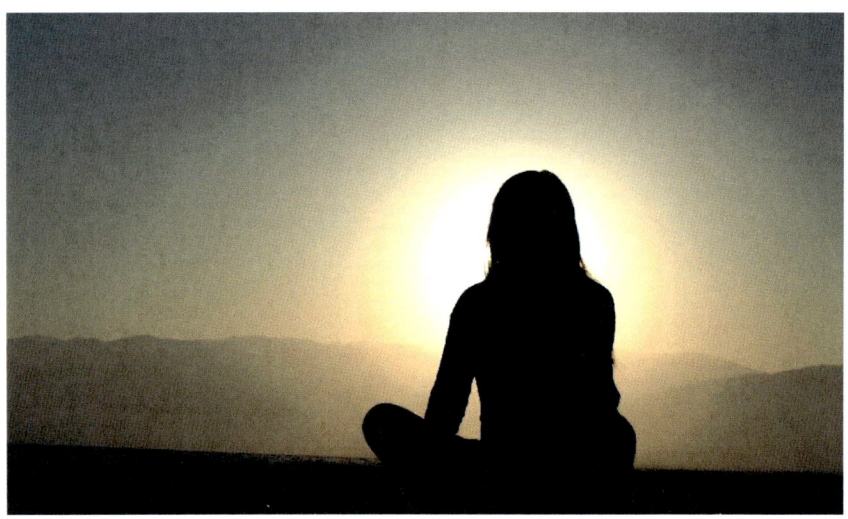

ENDNOTES

[i] President's Council on Sports, Fitness, and Nutrition. *Physical Activity Guidelines for Americans* 2nd Edition.

[ii] "The Big Picture: Checking Your Blood Glucose." diabetes.org. American Diabetes Association, (2019). May 2019.

[iii] The American Association of Clinical Endocrinologists and American College of Endocrinology on the Comprehensive Type 2 Diabetes Management Algorithm.

[iv] "Statistics About Diabetes." diabetes.org. American Diabetes Association, (2017). May 2019.

[v] *Harrison's Principles of Internal Medicine, 20e.* New York, NY: McGraw-Hill; 2018. (pg 2877)

[vi] *Harrison's Principles of Internal Medicine, 20e.* New York, NY: McGraw-Hill; 2018 (pg 2879)

[vii] *Harrison's Principles of Internal Medicine, 20e.* New York, NY: McGraw-Hill; 2018. (pg 2881)

[viii] U.S. Department of Health and Human Services and U.S. Department of Agriculture.

[ix] U.S. Department of Health and Human Services and U.S. Department of Agriculture.

[x] "Get Smart on Carb Counting." diabetes.org. American Diabetes Association, (2017). May 2019.

REFERENCES

Longo DL, Fauci AS, Kasper DL, Hauser SL, Jameson J, Loscalzo J. eds. *Harrison's Principles of Internal Medicine, 20e.* New York, NY: McGraw-Hill; 2018. Print.

Papadakis, Maxine A, Stephen J. McPhee, and Michael W. Rabow. *Current Medical Diagnosis & Treatment 2019.*, 2019. Print.

Pharmacologic Approaches to Glycemic Treatment: *Standards of Medical Care in Diabetes—2019* American Diabetes Association. Diabetes Care 2019 Jan; 42(Supplement 1): S90-S102.https://doi.org/10.2337/dc19-S009

President's Council on Sports, Fitness, and Nutrition. *Physical Activity Guidelines for Americans* 2nd Edition. https://www.hhs.gov/fitness/index.html

The American Association of Clinical Endocrinologists and American College of Endocrinology on the Comprehensive Type 2 Diabetes Management Algorithm. *2019 Executive Summary*. Endocrine Practice: January 2019, Vol. 25, No. 1, pp. 69-100.

U.S. Department of Health and Human Services and U.S. Department of Agriculture. *2015 – 2020 Dietary Guidelines for Americans*. 8th Edition. December 2015. https://health.gov/dietaryguidelines/2015/guidelines/.

www. diabetes.org. American Diabetes Association

GLOSSARY

BMI-Body Mass Index is a measure of fat based on height, weight, and gender. It can be determined by using the following equation: (weight/height$^{2)}$ x703)
Calorie- A unit used to measure the amount of energy in food.
Carbohydrate-One of the 3 major building blocks found in food. There are 3 types of carbohydrates: sugar, starch, and fiber.
Diabetes Type I- It is an autoimmune disease caused by destruction of the cells of the pancreas to the point that they will no longer produce insulin.
Diabetes Type II- Is described as disorder of "insulin resistance". The pancreas works harder to release more insulin to take extra glucose into the cells and over time cannot keep up.
Diabetic ketoacidosis (DKA)- A life-threatening condition caused by severely high glucose levels; typically seen in Type I diabetics and symptoms typically occur over a 24-hour time period
Endocrinologist-A doctor that specializes in metabolic disorders including diabetes.
ESRD-End stage renal disease, a condition where the kidneys stop working and machines (dialysis) perform the functions that the kidneys can no longer do.
Glucometer-A home measuring device used to test your glucose levels.
Glucose-A simple carbohydrate used by the body for energy.
Glycemic index- A system that measures how a food containing carbohydrate raises your blood sugar.
HgbA1c (glycated hemoglobin)-An average of your blood sugar over the last 3 months.
Hyperglycemia-Too much glucose in the blood stream; often caused by diabetes.
Hyperosmolar Hyperglycemic State-A life-threating condition caused by severely high glucose levels; typically seen in Type II diabetics and symptoms typically occur gradually over several weeks.
Hypoglycemia-Too low glucose in the blood stream; often caused by insulin therapy or other diabetic medications.
Insulin- A hormone made by the pancreas that is released when you eat foods containing carbohydrates; allowing the body to use glucose for energy.
Lancet- A sharp device used by diabetic patients to prick the finger to test their glucose with a glucometer.
Lipodystrophy- Visible lumps or small dents in the skin typically caused by injecting insulin at the same site daily.
Nephrologist- A doctor that specializes in the health of your kidneys.
Nephropathy-Disease of the kidneys.

Neuropathy-Disease of the nerves typically causing pain, numbness, and tingling.
Ophthalmologist-A doctor that specializes in eye health.
Pancreas-An organ located near the stomach that is part of your digestive system and makes insulin.
Podiatrist- A doctor that specializes in disease of the feet.
Post prandial glucose-Glucose reading taken 2 hours after the last meal was eaten.
Pre-diabetes- A condition where the glucose levels are high due to insulin resistance but not high enough to be classified as diabetes.
Retinal ischemia- A condition of the eye where the retina does not get enough blood supply
Retinopathy-Disease of the retina of the eyes
Syringe- A small tube with a needle placed on the end used for injecting insulin.
Vial-A glass container used to store liquid medication such as insulin.

APPENDIX

Glucose Monitoring Logs

Date	Fasting Glucose	2 Hour After Breakfast Glucose	Before Lunch Glucose	Before Dinner Glucose	Bedtime
Example 1/1/20					

Glucose Monitoring Logs

Date	Fasting Glucose	2 Hour After Breakfast Glucose	Before Lunch Glucose	Before Dinner Glucose	Bedtime

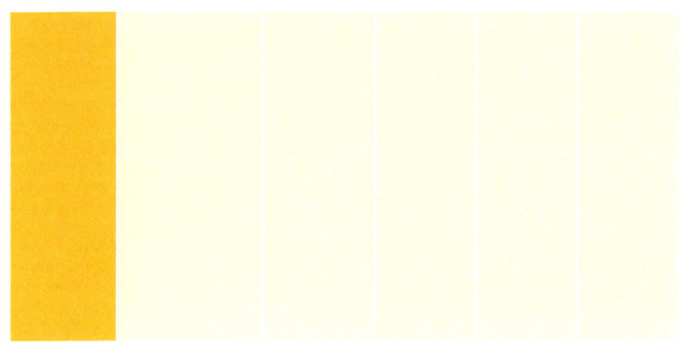

Glucose Monitoring Logs

Date	Fasting Glucose	2 Hour After Breakfast Glucose	Before Lunch Glucose	Before Dinner Glucose	Bedtime

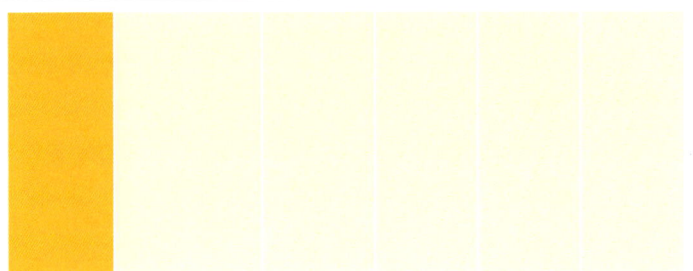

*All photos courtesy of Unsplash.com with credit to those listed below:

Sugar building blocks by Mae Mu
Salad bar by Dan Gold
Lab draw and woman during eye examination by Hush Naidoo
Woman on scale Photo i yunmai
Two women studying by Alissa De Leva
Glucometer by Kate
City runners by Martins Zemlickis
Grocery shopping by Hanson Lu
Pill box by Laurynas Mereckas
Syringe and apple by Sara Bakhshi
Breakfast by Jannis Brandt
Eye by v2osk
Heart and kidney model by Robina Weermeijer
Oatmeal by Alexandru Acea
Pancakes, eggs, and bacon by Gabriel Gurrola
Burrito bowl by Charles Koh
Burger and fries by Prudence Earl
Salmon by Caroline Attwood
Fried fish by Calvin Ma
Sunset by Dingzeyu Li

ABOUT THE AUTHOR

Dr. Ebony Raymond D.O. is a practicing internal medicine physician. She is practice owner of The Medical Institute for Wellness, a primary care clinic in Plano, TX. She has a B.S. in Kinesiology from Texas Christian University. She attended medical school at William Carey University College of Medicine and completed her internal medicine residency at Medical City Weatherford in July 2019. Her philosophy is built on 3 John 1:2 (NASB), *"Beloved, I pray that in all respects you may prosper and be in good health, just as your soul prospers."* This book in addition to her book, *"Rise and Grind to Shine Devotional: Biblical Truth for Victorious Living"* is part of her mission to ensure that everyone achieve total wellness in every aspect of their life including body, mind, and spirit.

For more information please visit her website at:
www.drebonyraymond.com

Follow on social media!
Instagram: @drebonyraymond
Twitter: @DrEbonyRaymond1
Facebook: www.facebook.com/ebony.raymond.33
YouTube: www.youtube.com/channel/UCYrjB3ZB6PSyFoQdTgVyjqA

Made in the USA
Coppell, TX
13 May 2020